THE MAGIC IN MICRODOSING: HOW PSILOCYBIN CAN IMPROVE YOUR LIFE

CHAPTER 1 INTRODUCTION

In recent years, there has been a growing interest in microdosing psilocybin, a practice that involves taking small, sub-perceptual doses of the psychedelic compound found in certain species of mushrooms. Microdosing has gained popularity as a way to experience the benefits of psilocybin without the intense psychedelic effects.

Psilocybin is a naturally occurring psychedelic compound found in over 200 species of mushrooms, most commonly in the Psilocybe genus. When consumed, psilocybin is converted into psilocin in the body, which acts on serotonin receptors in the brain to produce altered states of consciousness. Psilocybin has been used for centuries in various cultures for spiritual and medicinal purposes.

The use of psilocybin-containing mushrooms dates back to ancient times, with evidence of their use found in pre-Columbian Mesoamerica, where they were used in religious and healing ceremonies. Psilocybin mushrooms have also been

used in various cultures around the world for their spiritual and medicinal properties.

Despite the long history of psilocybin use, it wasn't until the mid-twentieth century that scientists began to study its effects. In the 1950s and 60s, researchers like Timothy Leary and Richard Alpert (later known as Ram Dass) conducted studies on the use of psilocybin for psychotherapy and spiritual exploration. However, with the rise of the counterculture movement and concerns about the potential risks of psychedelics, research into psilocybin was largely abandoned.

In recent years, however, there has been a renewed interest in psilocybin research. Advances in technology have made it easier to study the effects of psilocybin on the brain, and researchers have begun to explore its potential therapeutic benefits.

While recreational use of psilocybin mushrooms has been popular for decades, microdosing offers a new way to experience the benefits of psilocybin without the intense psychedelic experience. Microdosing involves taking small doses of psilocybin, usually one-tenth to one-twentieth of a typical recreational dose, on a regular basis. This practice is thought to produce subtle changes in mood, perception, and cognitive function, without the intense psychedelic effects.

The use of psilocybin for therapeutic purposes is still in its early stages, but initial studies have shown promising results. Psilocybin has been shown to reduce symptoms of depression and anxiety, and to improve cognitive function. In addition, studies have shown that psilocybin can produce mystical experiences, which have been linked to positive changes in personality, behavior, and overall well-being.

Despite the promising results of psilocybin research, there are still many questions that remain unanswered. Further research is needed to fully understand the effects of psilocybin, both in microdoses and in larger doses, and to explore its potential therapeutic uses.

In this book, we will explore the history, science, and potential benefits of microdosing psilocybin, as well as how to do so safely and effectively. We will also examine potential risks and side effects, and offer practical guidance for those interested in exploring microdosing as a tool for personal growth and healing.

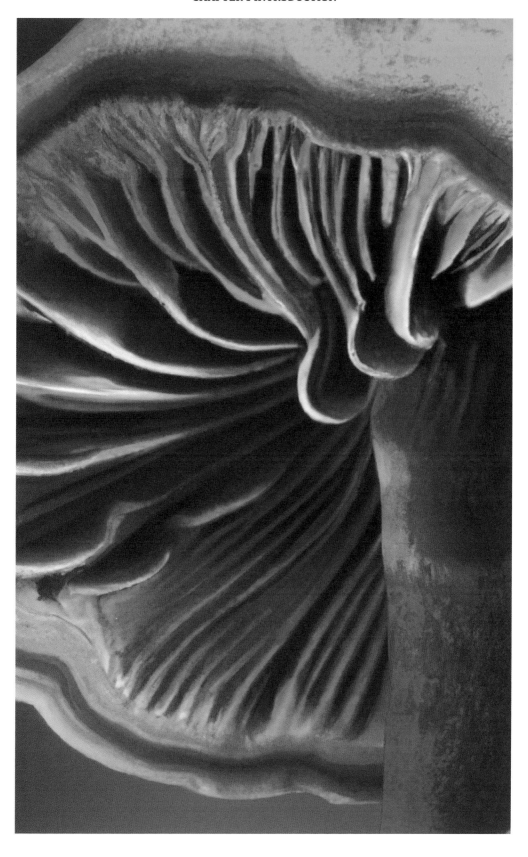

CHAPTER 2: UNDERSTANDING PSILOCYBIN

Psilocybin is a naturally occurring psychedelic compound found in over 200 species of mushrooms, most commonly in the Psilocybe genus. When consumed, psilocybin is converted into psilocin in the body, which acts on serotonin receptors in the brain to produce altered states of consciousness. Psilocybin has been used for centuries in various cultures for spiritual and medicinal purposes.

Psilocybin belongs to a class of drugs known as psychedelics, which produce profound changes in perception, thought, and mood. Other psychedelics include LSD, mescaline, and DMT. While the effects of each psychedelic are unique, they share certain similarities, such as producing changes in perception and enhancing introspection.

The chemical structure of psilocybin is similar to that of serotonin, a neurotransmitter that plays a role in regulating mood, appetite, and sleep. Psilocybin binds to serotonin receptors in the brain, which leads to increased activity in certain brain regions, including the default mode network (DMN). The DMN is a network of brain regions that are active during states of rest and mind-wandering, and are thought to be involved in self-referential thinking and autobiographical memory. When psilocybin is taken, the DMN is disrupted, leading to a breakdown in the sense of self and an increase in creative thinking.

The effects of psilocybin can be highly variable, depending on factors such as dose, setting, and individual differences. At low doses, psilocybin can produce feelings of relaxation and euphoria, while at higher doses, it can produce profound changes in perception, including visual hallucinations and alterations in time perception.

The subjective effects of psilocybin can also vary widely depending on the individual. Some people report feeling more connected to nature or a sense of universal oneness, while others report experiencing intense emotions or insights into their own lives.

Despite the powerful effects of psilocybin, it is generally considered to be safe, with a low risk of overdose or addiction. However, as with any drug, there are potential risks and side effects, particularly when taken in high doses or in unsafe environments.

In recent years, researchers have become increasingly interested in the potential therapeutic benefits of psilocybin. Studies have shown that psilocybin can be effective in treating depression, anxiety, addiction, and other mental health conditions. Additionally, psilocybin has been shown to enhance creativity, boost mood, and improve overall well-being.

While the therapeutic benefits of psilocybin are still being studied, it is clear that this compound has tremendous potential as a tool for personal growth and healing. In the following chapters, we will explore the benefits of microdosing psilocybin and how it can be used as a safe and effective means of exploring the benefits of this remarkable substance.

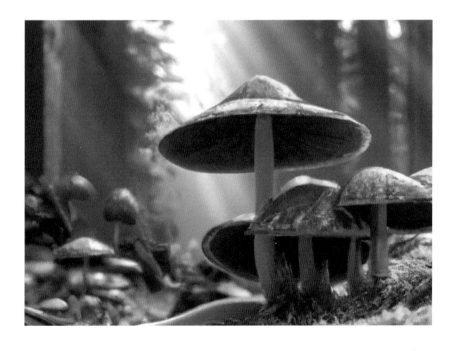

CHAPTER 3: BRIEF HISTORY OF HUMANS USING PSILOCYBIN

Humans have been using psilocybin-containing mushrooms for thousands of years, with evidence of their use dating back to prehistoric times. Psilocybin mushrooms have been used for a variety of purposes throughout history, ranging from spiritual and religious ceremonies to medicinal and recreational use.

One of the earliest known uses of psilocybin mushrooms was among indigenous tribes in Central and South America. The Mazatec people of Mexico have a long tradition of using psilocybin mushrooms in shamanic rituals, where they are consumed for their spiritual and medicinal properties. The use of psilocybin mushrooms in these cultures is often associated with healing, divination, and communication with the spirit world.

In addition to Central and South America, psilocybin mushrooms have also been used in other parts of the world. In Africa, the Khoisan people of the Kalahari Desert have used psilocybin mushrooms for generations, consuming them for their psychoactive effects during hunting trips and other rituals. In Europe, psilocybin mushrooms were used by ancient Greeks and Romans for their mind-altering properties.

During the 20th century, psilocybin mushrooms gained popularity among the counterculture movement of the 1960s and 1970s. The recreational use of psilocybin mushrooms became more widespread during this time, as people sought out new experiences and alternative forms of consciousness. However, the use of psilocybin mushrooms was made illegal in the United States in 1970, and remains illegal in many countries around the world.

Despite their illegal status, research into the potential therapeutic benefits of psilocybin mushrooms has continued. In recent years, there has been a renewed interest in psilocybin as a tool for personal growth and healing, and studies have shown promising results for its use in treating a variety of mental health conditions.

Today, psilocybin mushrooms are still used in some traditional cultures, and have also gained popularity as a tool for spiritual exploration, personal development, and recreational use. However, it is important to note that the possession and use of psilocybin mushrooms remains illegal in many countries, and can carry significant legal risks. It is also important to use caution when consuming psilocybin mushrooms, as they can produce powerful effects and can be potentially dangerous in certain situations.

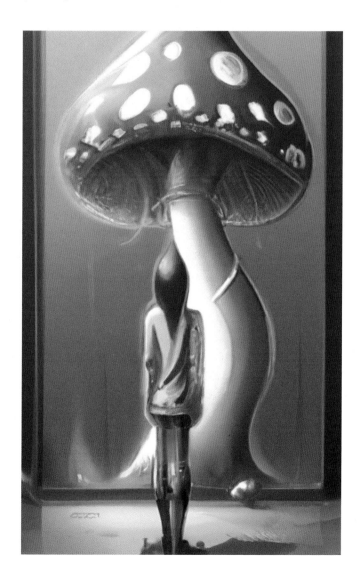

CHAPTER 4: THE BENEFITS OF MICRODOSING PSILOCYBIN

Microdosing psilocybin is the practice of consuming sub-perceptual doses of psilocybin mushrooms, typically every few days over a period of several weeks or months. While the effects of microdosing are much subtler than those of a full dose, many people have reported significant benefits from this practice.

Increased Creativity And Productivity

One of the most commonly reported benefits of microdosing psilocybin is an increase in creativity and productivity. Many people have reported that microdosing helps them to think more creatively, come up with new ideas, and be more productive in their work. This is likely due to the fact that psilocybin has been shown to increase connectivity in the brain, particularly in areas associated with creativity and problem-solving.

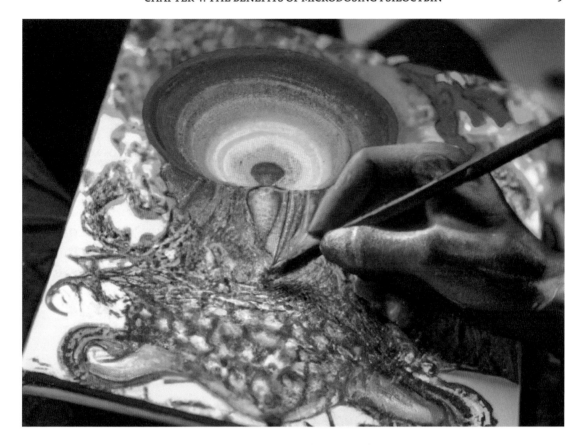

Improved Mood And Emotional Well-Being

Another benefit of microdosing psilocybin is an improvement in mood and emotional well-being. Psilocybin has been shown to have antidepressant and anti-anxiety effects, and many people report feeling more positive and less stressed after microdosing. This is likely due to psilocybin's ability to increase the production of serotonin, a neurotransmitter that plays a key role in regulating mood and emotions.

Increased Focus And Mindfulness

Microdosing psilocybin has also been reported to increase focus and mindfulness. Many people find that microdosing helps them to stay present in the moment, improve their attention span, and reduce distractibility. This may be due to psilocybin's ability to reduce activity in the default mode network, a network of brain regions that is active when our minds are at rest.

Reduced Pain And Inflammation

Recent research has suggested that psilocybin may have anti-inflammatory effects, which could be beneficial for people with conditions that involve chronic inflammation. In addition, some people have reported that microdosing psilocybin helps to reduce chronic pain, although more research is needed to understand the mechanisms behind this effect.

Increased Spiritual Awareness And Connection

Often people who microdose psilocybin report an increased sense of spiritual awareness and connection. Psilocybin has been used for centuries in traditional spiritual practices, and research has shown that it can increase feelings of awe and connection to nature. While this effect is subjective and difficult to measure, many people find that microdosing helps them to feel more connected to something greater than themselves.

The benefits of microdosing psilocybin are still being explored, and more research is needed to understand the full range of effects. Many people have reported significant benefits from this practice, and it has the potential to be a valuable tool for personal growth and healing.

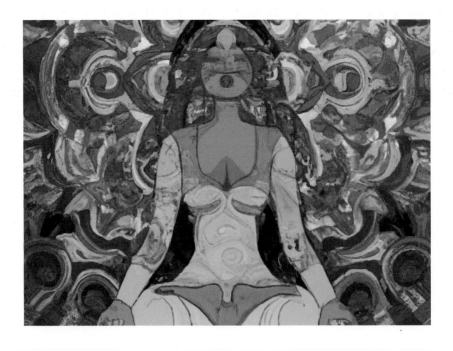

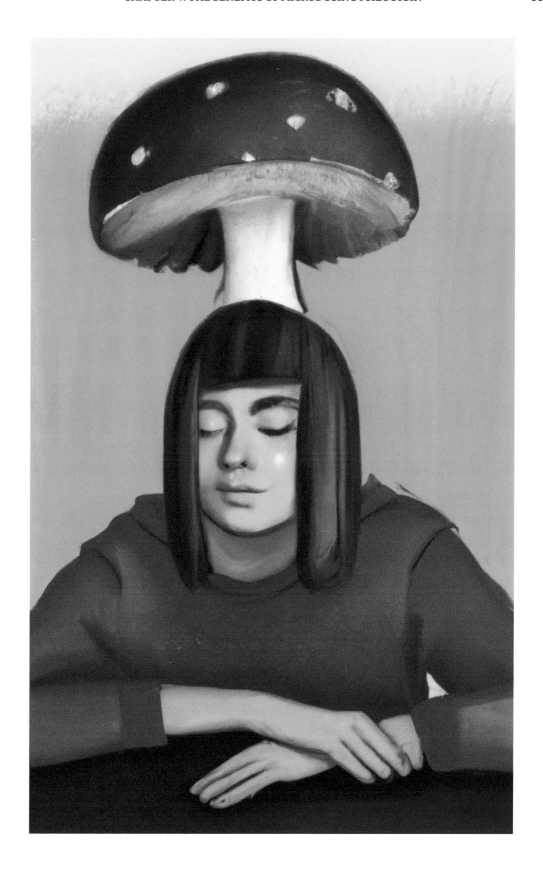

CHAPTER 5: THE SCIENCE OF MICRODOSING PSILOCYBIN

While the use of psilocybin for therapeutic and spiritual purposes dates back centuries, it is only in recent years that researchers have begun to explore the potential benefits of microdosing psilocybin. Here, we will examine the current state of scientific research on microdosing psilocybin, including what is known about its effects on the brain and body.

How Psilocybin Works In The Brain

Psilocybin is a psychedelic compound that works primarily by binding to serotonin receptors in the brain. Specifically, it binds to the 5-HT2A receptor, which is involved in the regulation of mood, perception, and cognition. When psilocybin binds to this receptor, it triggers a cascade of changes in the brain, including changes in blood flow, neural activity, and neurotransmitter levels.

One of the key effects of psilocybin is the reduction of activity in the default mode network (DMN), a network of brain regions that is active when our minds are at rest. This reduction in DMN activity is thought to underlie the profound changes in consciousness and perception that are associated with psilocybin use.

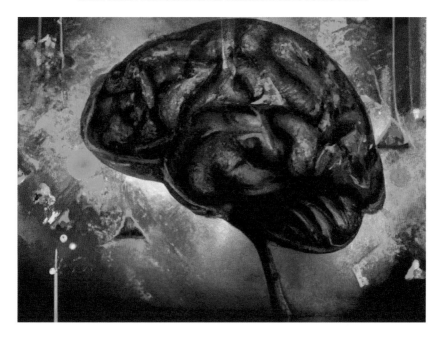

Microdosing And Brain Connectivity

Recent research has suggested that microdosing psilocybin may increase connectivity in the brain, particularly in areas associated with creativity and problem-solving. For example, a study published in the journal Psychopharmacology found that microdosing psilocybin increased functional connectivity between the medial prefrontal cortex and the posterior cingulate cortex, two brain regions that are part of the DMN.

Another study, published in the journal Frontiers in Psychology, found that microdosing psilocybin increased the diversity of brain activity in a sample of healthy volunteers. This increased diversity of activity was associated with improvements in mood, well-being, and cognitive flexibility.

Microdosing And Mood

Psilocybin has been shown to have antidepressant and anti-anxiety effects, and recent research has suggested that microdosing psilocybin may also have positive effects on mood and emotional well-being. A study published in the journal European Neuropsychopharmacology found that microdosing psilocybin led to improvements in depression and anxiety symptoms in a sample of people with treatment-resistant depression.

Another study, published in the Journal of Psychopharmacology, found that microdosing psilocybin led to improvements in emotional regulation and mindfulness in a sample of healthy volunteers.

Microdosing And Pain

While the effects of microdosing psilocybin on pain are not yet well understood, recent research has suggested that psilocybin may have anti-inflammatory effects. A study published in the journal Scientific Reports found that psilocybin reduced inflammation in a sample of mice with acute pancreatitis.

Another study, published in the journal Psychopharmacology, found that psilocybin reduced the perception of pain in a sample of healthy volunteers. However, more research is needed to understand the mechanisms behind this effect.

Microdosing And Spirituality

Microdosing psilocybin has been associated with increases in spiritual awareness and connection. A study published in the journal Frontiers in Psychology found that microdosing psilocybin increased feelings of awe and connection to nature in a sample of healthy volunteers.

Another study, published in the Journal of Psychopharmacology, found that psilocybin increased mystical experiences and feelings of unity in a sample of people with treatment-resistant depression.

While the scientific research on microdosing psilocybin is still in its early stages, the existing evidence suggests that this practice may have a range of positive effects on the brain and behavior.

As the research on microdosing psilocybin continues to grow, it will be important to gain a deeper understanding of its potential benefits, risks, and appropriate use. By staying informed and responsible, individuals may be able to harness the positive effects of microdosing psilocybin for personal growth and well-being.

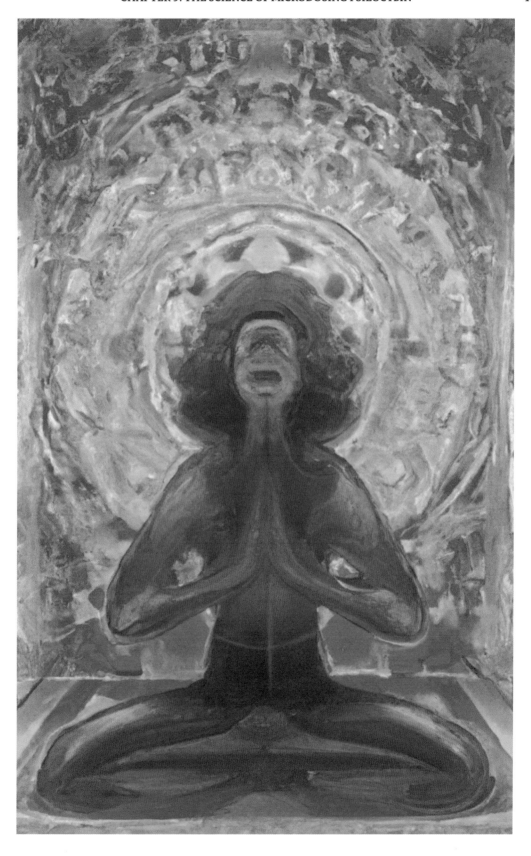

CHAPTER 6: THE THERAPEUTIC POTENTIAL OF MICRODOSING PSILOCYBIN

In recent years, researchers have begun to explore the potential therapeutic benefits of microdosing psilocybin, with promising results. Here, we will examine the current state of scientific research on the therapeutic potential of microdosing psilocybin, including its potential use in treating mental health conditions such as depression, anxiety, and addiction.

Microdosing And Depression

Depression is a common mental health condition that affects millions of people worldwide. While traditional treatments such as antidepressant medications and psychotherapy are effective for many people, some individuals may not respond well to these treatments or may experience significant side effects.

Recent research has suggested that microdosing psilocybin may have antidepressant effects. A study published in the journal European Neuropsychopharmacology found that microdosing psilocybin led to significant improvements in depression symptoms in a sample of people with treatment-resistant depression.

Another study, published in the journal Frontiers in Psychiatry, found that microdosing psilocybin improved emotional processing and cognitive flexibility in a sample of people with major depressive disorder.

Microdosing And Anxiety

Anxiety is another common mental health condition that can have a significant impact on a person's quality of life. While traditional treatments such as anti-anxiety medications and cognitive-behavioral therapy are effective for many people, some individuals may not respond well to these treatments or may experience significant side effects.

Recent research has suggested that microdosing psilocybin may have anti-anxiety effects. A study published in the journal Psychopharmacology found that microdosing psilocybin led to significant improvements in anxiety symptoms in a sample of people with social anxiety disorder.

Another study, published in the journal Scientific Reports, found that psilocybin reduced fear and anxiety in a sample of mice. While more research is needed to understand the effects of microdosing psilocybin on anxiety in humans, these early results are promising.

Microdosing And Addiction

Addiction is a complex mental health condition that can be difficult to treat using traditional methods. While medications and therapy can be effective for some people, others may require more intensive or specialized treatment.

Recent research has suggested that microdosing psilocybin may have potential as a treatment for addiction. A study published in the journal Journal of Psychopharmacology found that psilocybin-assisted therapy led to significant reductions in alcohol consumption in a sample of people with alcohol use disorder.

Another study, published in the journal ACS Pharmacology & Translational Science, found that psilocybin reduced the subjective effects of nicotine in a sample of smokers. While more research is needed to understand the mechanisms behind these effects, these early results suggest that microdosing psilocybin may have potential as a treatment for addiction.

Microdosing And Ptsd

Post-traumatic stress disorder (PTSD) is a mental health condition that can develop after a person experiences or witnesses a traumatic event. While traditional treatments such as psychotherapy and medications can be effective for some people, others may require additional or alternative treatments.

Recent research has suggested that microdosing psilocybin may have potential as a treatment for PTSD. A study published in the journal Frontiers in Psychiatry found that microdosing psilocybin led to significant improvements in PTSD symptoms in a sample of people with PTSD.

Another study, published in the journal ACS Pharmacology & Translational Science, found that psilocybin reduced fear in a sample of mice with PTSD-like symptoms. While more research is needed to understand the effects of microdosing psilocybin on PTSD in humans, these early results are promising.

Overall, the existing research suggests that microdosing psilocybin has the potential to offer numerous benefits for various conditions and situations. It may help alleviate symptoms of depression, anxiety, and other mental health disorders, as well as enhance creativity, cognitive function, and emotional regulation. However, it's important to note that psilocybin is still classified as a Schedule I drug in many countries.

CHAPTER 7: HOW TO MICRODOSE PSILOCYBIN SAFELY AND EFFECTIVELY

Microdosing psilocybin can offer a range of potential benefits, but it's important to approach this practice safely and responsibly. Here, we will discuss some key considerations to keep in mind when starting a microdosing regimen, including dosing guidelines, preparation, and potential risks.

Dosage Guidelines

One of the most important considerations when microdosing psilocybin is determining the appropriate dosage. A microdose is typically defined as a sub-perceptual amount of psilocybin, meaning that the user does not experience any psychedelic effects. The exact dose that constitutes a microdose can vary depending on a variety of factors, including individual body chemistry, tolerance, and the specific strain of psilocybin used.

As a general rule, a microdose of psilocybin is considered to be between 0.1 and 0.5 grams of dried mushrooms, or between 5 and 20 milligrams of pure psilocybin extract. However, it's important to start with a very low dose and gradually increase the amount over time as needed. It's also important to avoid taking too much, as this can lead to unwanted psychedelic effects.

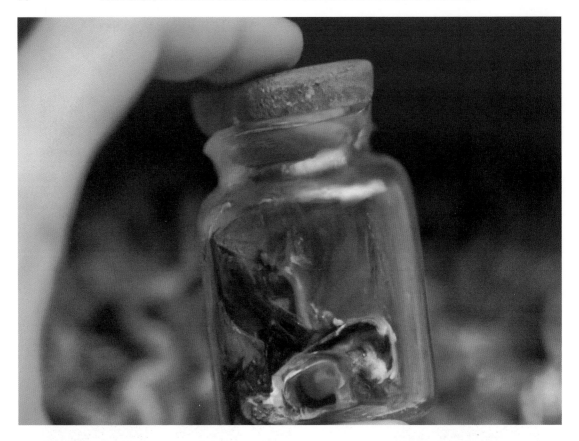

Preparation

Before beginning a microdosing regimen, it's important to prepare both physically and mentally. This can involve creating a comfortable and safe environment in which to take the microdose, as well as preparing oneself emotionally for any potential effects.

It's also important to choose a high-quality source of psilocybin, whether through purchasing dried mushrooms or obtaining a pure psilocybin extract from a reputable source. Ensure that the psilocybin is stored properly, as exposure to heat, light, and moisture can degrade the substance and reduce its potency.

Potential Risks

While microdosing psilocybin is generally considered safe, there are some potential risks to keep in mind. These can include:

- Psychotic episodes: While rare, some individuals may experience

psychotic episodes or other negative psychological effects when taking psilocybin.
- Physical side effects: Psilocybin can cause nausea, vomiting, and other physical symptoms in some individuals.
- Interactions with other medications: Psilocybin can interact with certain medications, including antidepressants and antipsychotics.

It's important to be aware of these potential risks and to consult with a healthcare professional before beginning a microdosing regimen, particularly if you have any underlying medical conditions or are taking other medications.

Best Practices

To ensure a safe and effective microdosing experience, it's important to follow some best practices:
- Start with a very low dose and gradually increase as needed.
- Take the microdose in a comfortable and safe environment.
- Keep a journal or record of your experiences, including any effects you may have felt.
- Take regular breaks from microdosing to avoid developing a tolerance or dependence.
- Consult with a healthcare professional if you have any underlying medical conditions or are taking other medications.

Choosing A Dosage Regimen

There are several different dosage regimens that can be used when microdosing psilocybin. Some people prefer to take a microdose every day, while others prefer to take a larger dose once a week or every other week. There is no one "right" dosage regimen, and it's important to experiment and find what works best for you.

It's also important to keep in mind that psilocybin can have a cumulative effect over time, meaning that the benefits may increase with continued use. However, it's also important to take breaks from microdosing to avoid building up tolerance and potential negative effects.

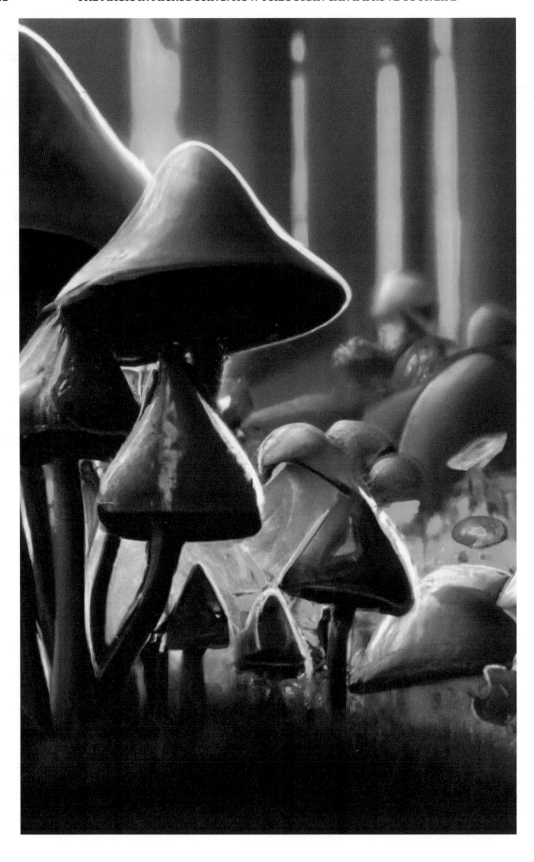

CHAPTER 8: POTENTIAL RISKS AND SIDE EFFECTS OF MICRODOSING PSILOCYBIN

While microdosing psilocybin can offer many benefits, it is important to consider the potential risks and side effects before deciding to try it. Although research suggests that microdosing is generally safe, it is not without risks, especially if not done properly. It is important to understand these risks and side effects and take steps to minimize them.

One of the primary risks associated with microdosing psilocybin is the potential for experiencing a bad trip. A bad trip is a negative psychedelic experience that can be caused by a number of factors, including taking too high of a dose, being in an uncomfortable or unfamiliar environment, or having a pre-existing mental health condition. It is important to start with a low dose and gradually increase it to minimize the risk of a bad trip. Additionally, it is important to only microdose in a comfortable and safe environment, with people you trust.

Another potential risk of microdosing is the potential for interactions with other medications or supplements. If you are taking any prescription medications or supplements, it is important to speak with a healthcare provider before starting to microdose. Psilocybin can interact with certain medications, such as antidepressants, and can have dangerous side effects when combined with them.

One of the most common side effects of microdosing psilocybin is increased anxiety. While some individuals report reduced anxiety as a benefit of microdosing, others may experience an increase in anxiety, especially if they are prone to anxiety. It is important to monitor your emotional state closely while microdosing and seek support if you experience increased anxiety.

Other potential side effects of microdosing psilocybin can include headaches, nausea, and increased heart rate. These side effects are generally mild and subside on their own within a few hours. However, if you experience any severe or prolonged side effects, it is important to seek medical attention immediately.

It is important to note that psilocybin is still illegal in many parts of the world. While some countries decriminalized or legalized psilocybin for medical or research purposes, it is still considered a Schedule I substance in many countries, which means that it is illegal to possess, use, or distribute. It is important to understand the legal status of psilocybin in your area before deciding to microdose.

Overall, while microdosing psilocybin can offer many potential benefits, it is important to be aware of the potential risks and side effects. It is important to start with a low dose, microdose in a safe and comfortable environment, and seek medical advice if you are taking other medications or supplements. If you experience any negative side effects, it is important to stop microdosing immediately and seek medical attention if necessary.

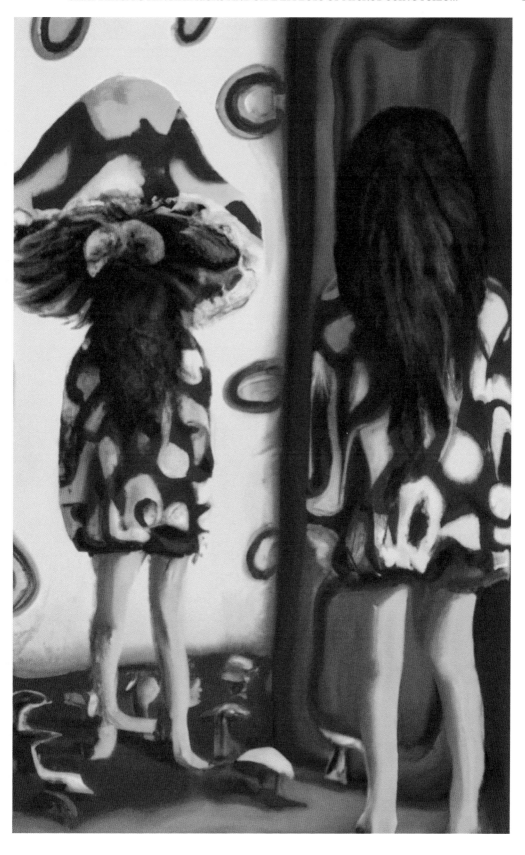

CHAPTER 9: MICRODOSING PSILOCYBIN - HOW TO GET STARTED

I f you have decided to try microdosing psilocybin, there are some important steps to take to ensure that you do it safely and effectively. Here are some guidelines to help you get started:

Do Your Research

Before starting to microdose, it is important to educate yourself about psilocybin and microdosing. Read books, articles, and scientific studies to learn about the potential benefits and risks of microdosing. Make sure you are informed about the legal status of psilocybin in your area, and seek advice from a healthcare provider if you have any medical conditions or are taking any medications.

Obtain High-Quality Psilocybin

It is important to obtain high-quality psilocybin from a reputable source. This can be in the form of mushrooms or a psilocybin extract. If you are obtaining psilocybin mushrooms, it is important to know how to identify them and ensure that they are safe to consume. If you are obtaining a psilocybin extract, make sure that it is from a reputable supplier and that it has been tested for purity and potency.

Start With A Low Dose

Start with a low dose when you first begin to microdose. A typical starting dose is around 0.1-0.3 grams of dried mushrooms, or 1-3 micrograms of psilocybin extract. This low dose allows you to test your sensitivity to psilocybin and helps you to avoid potential negative side effects.

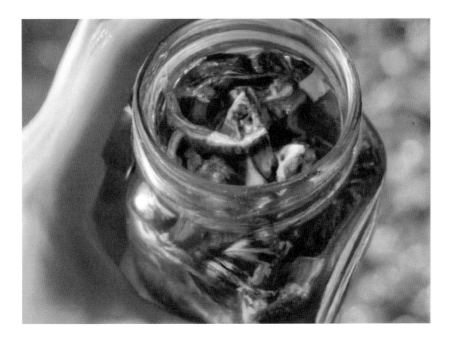

Develop A Dosing Schedule

Develop a dosing schedule that works for you. Some individuals choose to microdose every other day, while others choose to microdose every three or four days. It is important to maintain a consistent schedule to avoid tolerance and to monitor the effects of microdosing over time.

Keep A Journal

Keeping a journal of your microdosing experiences can be a helpful tool for monitoring your progress and noting any effects or changes you experience. It can be useful to record the time and dose of each microdose, as well as any physical or emotional effects you experience.
Set intentions: Before each microdose, it can be helpful to set intentions for what you hope to achieve or experience. This can help you to stay focused and mindful during the microdosing experience.

Create A Supportive Environment

It is important to create a supportive and comfortable environment for your microdosing experiences. Choose a quiet and safe space, and surround yourself with supportive and trusted people. Turn off your phone and other distractions to help you stay focused.

Be Patient

The effects of microdosing can take time to become noticeable, and the benefits may not be immediate or obvious. It is important to be patient and persistent with your microdosing practice, and to monitor your progress over time.

Overall, microdosing psilocybin can be a powerful tool for personal growth, creativity, and wellness. By following these guidelines and taking a cautious and mindful approach, you can safely and effectively incorporate microdosing into your daily routine.

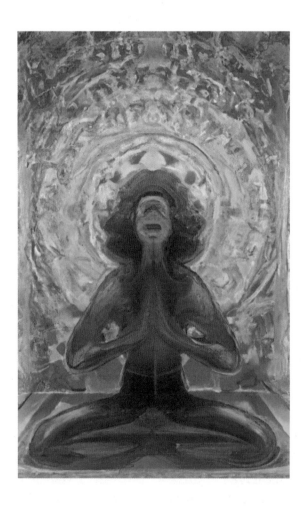

CHAPTER 10: CONCLUSION

In recent years, microdosing psilocybin has gained popularity as a potential tool for enhancing creativity, increasing focus and productivity, and promoting emotional well-being. While there is still much to learn about the effects of psilocybin, there is a growing body of research that suggests that microdosing may offer significant benefits for certain individuals.

One of the primary benefits of microdosing is the potential to enhance creativity and cognitive function. Many people report increased creativity and a greater ability to focus on tasks while microdosing, which may be due to changes in brain activity and connectivity.

Another potential benefit of microdosing is its ability to improve emotional well-being. Some studies have found that microdosing can reduce symptoms of anxiety and depression, and improve mood and emotional stability. This may be due to the way that psilocybin interacts with serotonin receptors in the brain.

In addition to these benefits, microdosing psilocybin may also have therapeutic potential for certain individuals. Research has shown that psilocybin may be effective in treating conditions such as anxiety, depression, and addiction, and may also have potential in treating other mental health disorders.

While microdosing psilocybin may offer many potential benefits, it is important to remember that it is not a cure-all solution, and should not be used as a substitute for professional medical treatment. It is also important to use caution when experimenting with psilocybin, as it can have potential risks and side effects.

If you are considering microdosing psilocybin, it is important to educate yourself about the substance and to approach it with caution and mindfulness. Start with a low dose, develop a consistent dosing schedule, and create a supportive and comfortable environment for your microdosing experiences. Keep a journal to track your progress and monitor any effects or changes you experience.

Overall, microdosing psilocybin has the potential to offer significant benefits for those who use it mindfully and with caution. With further research and education, it may become a valuable tool for enhancing creativity, promoting emotional well-being, and treating certain mental health conditions.

References

Understanding Psilocybin
1. Nichols DE. Psychedelics. Pharmacol Rev. 2016;68(2):264-355. doi:10.1124/pr.115.011478
2. Carhart-Harris RL, Nutt DJ. Serotonin and brain function: a tale of two receptors. J Psychopharmacol. 2017;31(9):1091-1120. doi:10.1177/0269881117714399

Brief History of Humans Using Psilocybin
1. McKenna T. Food of the Gods: The Search for the Original Tree of Knowledge: A Radical History of Plants, Drugs, and Human Evolution. Bantam; 1993.
2. Stamets P. Psilocybin Mushrooms of the World: An Identification Guide. Ten Speed Press; 1996.

The Benefits of Microdosing Psilocybin
1. Fadiman J, Korb S. Microdosing Psychedelics: A Practical Guide to Upgrade Your Life. Sounds True; 2019.
2. Anderson T, Petranker R, Rosenbaum D, et al. Microdosing psychedelics: personality, mental health, and creativity differences in microdosers. Psychopharmacology (Berl). 2019;236(2):731-740. doi:10.1007/s00213-018-5077-4

The Science of Microdosing Psilocybin
1. Hutten NRPW, Mason NL, Dolder PC, Kuypers KPC. Motives and side-effects of microdosing with psychedelics among users. Int J Neuropsychopharmacol. 2019;22(7):426-434. doi:10.1093/ijnp/pyz028
2. Prochazkova L, Lippelt DP, Colzato LS, Kuchar M, Sjoerds Z, Hommel B. Exploring the effect of microdosing psychedelics on creativity in an open-label natural setting. Psychopharmacology (Berl). 2018;235(12):3401-3413. doi:10.1007/s00213-018-5049-8

The Therapeutic Potential of Microdosing Psilocybin

1. Garcia-Romeu A, Davis AK, Erowid F, Erowid E, Griffiths RR, Johnson MW. Cessation and reduction in alcohol consumption and misuse after psychedelic use. J Psychopharmacol. 2019;33(10):1088-1101. doi:10.1177/0269881119857204

2. Polito V, Stevenson RJ. A systematic study of microdosing psychedelics. PLoS One. 2019;14(2):e0211023. doi:10.1371/journal.pone.0211023

Potential Risks and Side Effects of Microdosing Psilocybin

1. Yensen R, Doblin R. The use of LSD and other hallucinogens in psychotherapy and for personal growth. J Transpers Psychol. 1994;26(1):1-27.

2. Bershad AK, Schepers ST, Bremmer MP, et al. Acute subjective and behavioral effects of microdoses of lysergic acid diethylamide in healthy human volunteers.

Printed in Great Britain
by Amazon

37049149R00021